The Simple
DIVERTICULITIS
COOKBOOK 101

Adeola Ganiu

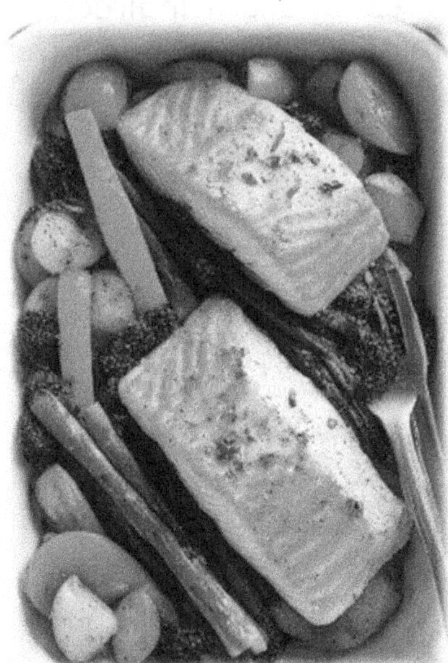

Dedication

To everyone who is cooking their way to a better and healthier life.

Table of Contents

INTRODUCTION

ccording to the National Institute of Diabetes and Digestive and Kidney Diseases (NIDDK), diverticulitis affects about 200,000 people in the United States annually. While the prevalence of diverticulosis, the condition of having diverticula in the colon, increases with age, not everyone with diverticulosis develops diverticulitis. However, when inflammation or infection does occur, it can lead to severe pain, fever, and other serious complications. Effective management of diverticulitis is crucial to preventing these flare-ups and maintaining a good quality of life.

The first chapter of this book explores the nature of diverticulitis, its causes, symptoms, and the importance of diet in managing this condition. The rest of book provides a collection of carefully curated recipes designed to be gentle on the digestive system while ensuring nutritional balance and delicious flavors. This two-pronged approach aims to empower you with the knowledge and tools needed to manage diverticulitis effectively.

1. UNDERSTANDING DIVERTICULITIS

What is Diverticulitis?

Diverticulitis is a condition where small pouches (diverticula) in the wall of the colon become inflamed or infected. Symptoms can range from mild discomfort to severe pain, and in some cases, complications can arise. While the exact cause of diverticulitis is not fully understood, diet plays a crucial role in both preventing flare-ups and managing symptoms when they occur.

How Diet Affects Diverticulitis

The foods you eat can either contribute to the inflammation of diverticula or help in soothing and healing your digestive tract. A diet rich in fiber, for example, can promote regular bowel movements and reduce the risk of diverticulitis, while certain foods may exacerbate symptoms during an acute episode. This cookbook aims to guide you through these dietary nuances, offering recipes tailored to each phase of diverticulitis management.

Causes and Symptoms

<u>**Causes**</u>

The exact cause of diverticulitis is not entirely understood, but several factors are believed to contribute to the development of this condition:

Low-Fiber Diet: A diet low in fiber can lead to constipation and increased pressure in the colon, which may cause diverticula to form.

Aging: As people age, the walls of the colon can become weaker and more susceptible to the formation of diverticula.

Genetics: There may be a hereditary component, as diverticulitis can run in families.

Lack of Exercise: Sedentary lifestyles are associated with a higher risk of developing diverticulitis.

Obesity: Being overweight can increase the likelihood of diverticulitis.

Smoking: Smoking has been linked to a higher risk of diverticulitis.

<u>**Symptoms**</u>

The symptoms of diverticulitis can vary in severity and may include:

Abdominal Pain: Typically located in the lower left side of the abdomen, the pain can be severe and persistent.

Fever: A sign of infection, fever often accompanies diverticulitis.

Nausea and Vomiting: These symptoms can occur if the infection or inflammation is severe.

Changes in Bowel Habits: This can include constipation, diarrhea, or a combination of both.

Bloating and Gas: Discomfort and bloating can occur due to digestive disturbances.

Loss of Appetite: A reduced desire to eat is common during a flare-up.

Managing Diverticulitis with Diet

Diet plays a crucial role in both the prevention and management of diverticulitis. Understanding how to adjust your eating habits can help reduce the risk of flare-ups and manage symptoms effectively.

Prevention

High-Fiber Diet: Consuming a diet rich in fiber is key to preventing diverticulitis. Fiber helps soften stool and promotes regular bowel movements, reducing the pressure on the colon. Good sources of fiber include fruits, vegetables, whole grains, and legumes.

Hydration: Drinking plenty of water helps fiber work more effectively and prevents constipation.

Regular Meals: Eating regular meals can help maintain consistent bowel movements.

During a Flare-Up

Clear Liquid Diet: During an acute attack, a clear liquid diet can help rest the digestive system. This includes broths, clear juices, and gelatin.

Low-Fiber Diet: As symptoms improve, transitioning to a low-fiber diet can ease the digestive process. Foods like white rice, white bread, and cooked vegetables are recommended.

Gradual Introduction of Fiber: Once symptoms have fully subsided, gradually reintroducing fiber into the diet is important to avoid constipation and prevent future flare-ups.

Long-Term Management

Consistent Fiber Intake: Maintaining a high-fiber diet long-term is crucial. Incorporating a variety of fiber-rich foods can help keep the digestive system functioning well.

Balanced Diet: Ensuring a balanced diet with adequate nutrients supports overall health and digestive function.

Avoiding Trigger Foods: Some individuals may find that certain foods trigger symptoms. Common culprits include nuts, seeds, and popcorn, although this varies from person to person.

Dietary Phases

The Diverticulitis Diet is typically broken down into different phases, each designed to support healing and prevent flare-ups.

Dietary Phases

1. Clear Liquid Diet

Purpose: To rest the digestive system during an acute diverticulitis flare-up, reduce inflammation, and prevent complications.

Duration: Usually 1-3 days, depending on the severity of symptoms and as advised by a healthcare provider.

Foods Allowed:

- Water
- Clear broths (chicken, beef, or vegetable)
- Clear juices without pulp (apple, cranberry, grape)
- Gelatin (without added fruit)
- Popsicles (without fruit pieces or pulp)
- Tea or coffee (without cream or milk)

Foods to Avoid:

- Solid foods
- Dairy products
- Alcohol and caffeinated beverages (if they cause discomfort)

2. Low-Fiber Diet

Purpose: To transition the digestive system from a clear liquid diet to solid foods gently, reducing the risk of irritation and promoting gradual recovery.

Duration: Typically 3-7 days or until symptoms improve, as directed by a healthcare provider.

Foods Allowed:

- Low-fiber cereals and refined grains (white bread, white rice, pasta)

- Cooked or canned fruits without skin or seeds (applesauce, peaches, pears)
- Cooked vegetables without skin (carrots, green beans, potatoes)
- Lean proteins (skinless chicken, fish, eggs)
- Dairy products (milk, yogurt, cheese, if tolerated)

Foods to Avoid:

- High-fiber foods (whole grains, raw vegetables, legumes)
- Foods with seeds and nuts
- Spicy and fatty foods

3. Gradual Introduction of Fiber

Purpose: To reintroduce fiber into the diet slowly, promoting regular bowel movements and preventing future flare-ups.

Duration: Gradual reintroduction over several weeks, monitoring for any recurrence of symptoms.

Foods to Reintroduce Gradually:

- Whole grains (oats, brown rice, whole wheat bread)
- Raw fruits and vegetables (start with small portions)
- Legumes and beans (lentils, chickpeas)
- Nuts and seeds (if tolerated)

Tips for Gradual Introduction:

- Start with small portions and increase gradually.
- Incorporate one new high-fiber food at a time.
- Drink plenty of water to help fiber move through the digestive system.
- Pay attention to your body's response and adjust as necessary.

4. High-Fiber Maintenance Diet

Purpose: To maintain digestive health and prevent the recurrence of diverticulitis by promoting regular, healthy bowel movements.

Long-Term Foods to Include:

- High-fiber fruits (apples, pears, berries)

- Vegetables (broccoli, Brussels sprouts, carrots)
- Whole grains (quinoa, barley, whole wheat pasta)
- Legumes (black beans, kidney beans, lentils)
- Nuts and seeds (chia seeds, flaxseeds, almonds, if tolerated)

General Tips for Maintenance:

- Aim for a daily fiber intake of 25-30 grams.
- Stay hydrated with at least 8 cups of water per day.
- Incorporate a variety of fiber sources to ensure a balanced diet.
- Monitor for any potential trigger foods and adjust intake accordingly.

2. BREAKFAST RECIPES

Berry Fiber Blast Smoothie

Servings: 2   **Calories:** 180 per serving

Ingredients:

1 cup blueberries

1 cup strawberries

1 banana

1 cup spinach

1 tablespoon chia seeds

1 cup almond milk

1 tablespoon honey (optional)

Instructions:

Place all ingredients in a blender.

Blend until smooth.

Pour into glasses and serve immediately.

Green Detox Smoothie

Servings: 2   **Calories:** 150 per serving

Ingredients:

1 cucumber, peeled and chopped

1 green apple, cored and chopped

1 cup kale, stems removed

1/2 lemon, juiced

1 inch ginger, peeled

1 cup coconut water

Instructions:

Combine all ingredients in a blender.

Blend until smooth.

Serve chilled.

Carrot-Apple Juice

Servings: 2   **Calories:** 120 per serving

Ingredients:

3 large carrots

2 apples

1 inch ginger, peeled

1/2 lemon, juiced

Instructions:

Juice all ingredients using a juicer.

Stir to combine.

Serve immediately.

Oatmeal with Fresh Fruits

Servings: 2   **Calories:** 220 per serving

Ingredients:

1 cup rolled oats

2 cups water or almond milk

1/2 cup blueberries

1/2 cup sliced strawberries

1 tablespoon honey

Instructions:

In a pot, bring water or almond milk to a boil.

Add oats and reduce heat to simmer.

Cook for 5-7 minutes, stirring occasionally.

Serve with fresh fruits and honey on top.

Yogurt Parfait with Berries

Servings: 2   **Calories:** 200 per serving

Ingredients:

2 cups Greek yogurt

1 cup mixed berries (blueberries, strawberries, raspberries)

2 tablespoons granola (optional)

1 tablespoon honey

Instructions:

Layer yogurt, berries, and granola in a glass.

Drizzle with honey.

Serve immediately.

Soft Scrambled Eggs with Spinach

Servings: 2   **Calories:** 160 per serving

Ingredients:

4 large eggs

1/4 cup milk

1 cup fresh spinach, chopped

Salt and pepper to taste

1 tablespoon olive oil

Instructions:

In a bowl, whisk together eggs, milk, salt, and pepper.

Heat olive oil in a skillet over medium heat.

Add spinach and cook until wilted.

Pour in the egg mixture.

Cook, stirring gently, until eggs are just set.

Serve immediately.

Whole Grain Pancakes

Servings: 4   **Calories:** 180 per serving

Ingredients:

1 cup whole wheat flour

1 tablespoon baking powder

1/4 teaspoon salt

1 cup almond milk

1 egg

2 tablespoons honey

1 teaspoon vanilla extract

1 tablespoon coconut oil

Instructions:

In a bowl, mix flour, baking powder, and salt.

In another bowl, whisk together milk, egg, honey, and vanilla.

Combine wet and dry ingredients, mixing until smooth.

Heat coconut oil in a skillet over medium heat.

Pour batter into the skillet, forming pancakes.

Cook until bubbles form on the surface, then flip and cook until golden.

Serve with fresh fruit or syrup.

Quinoa Breakfast Bowl

Servings: 2   **Calories:** 220 per serving

Ingredients:

1 cup cooked quinoa

1/2 cup almond milk

1 banana, sliced

1/4 cup chopped nuts (almonds, walnuts)

1 tablespoon honey

Instructions:

In a bowl, combine cooked quinoa and almond milk.

Top with banana slices and nuts.

Drizzle with honey.

Serve warm.

Avocado Toast on Whole Wheat Bread

Servings: 2   **Calories:** 210 per serving

Ingredients:

2 slices whole wheat bread

1 ripe avocado

1 tablespoon lemon juice

Salt and pepper to taste

1/4 teaspoon red pepper flakes (optional)

Instructions:

Toast the whole wheat bread.

In a bowl, mash the avocado with lemon juice, salt, and pepper.

Spread the avocado mixture on the toasted bread.

Sprinkle with red pepper flakes if desired.

Serve immediately.

Baked Apples with Cinnamon

Servings: 2   **Calories:** 150 per serving

Ingredients:

2 apples, cored

1 tablespoon honey

1 teaspoon cinnamon

1/4 cup chopped nuts (optional)

Instructions:

Preheat the oven to 350°F (175°C).

Place the cored apples in a baking dish.

Drizzle with honey and sprinkle with cinnamon.

Fill the centers with chopped nuts if using.

Bake for 20-25 minutes, until apples are tender.

Serve warm.

Spinach and Tomato Omelette

Servings: 2   **Calories:** 170 per serving

Ingredients:

4 large eggs

1/4 cup milk

1 cup fresh spinach, chopped

1/2 cup cherry tomatoes, halved

Salt and pepper to taste

1 tablespoon olive oil

Instructions:

In a bowl, whisk together eggs, milk, salt, and pepper.

Heat olive oil in a skillet over medium heat.

Add spinach and tomatoes, cooking until spinach is wilted.

Pour in the egg mixture.

Cook until the eggs are set, then fold in half.

Serve immediately.

Apple Cinnamon Overnight Oats

Servings: 2   **Calories:** 230 per serving

Ingredients:

1 cup rolled oats

1 cup almond milk

1 apple, diced

1 tablespoon honey

1 teaspoon cinnamon

Instructions:

In a jar or container, combine oats, almond milk, apple, honey, and cinnamon.

Mix well, cover, and refrigerate overnight.

In the morning, stir and serve cold or warmed up.

Cottage Cheese and Pineapple Bowl

Servings: 2   **Calories:** 180 per serving

Ingredients:

1 cup low-fat cottage cheese

1 cup pineapple chunks

1 tablespoon honey

1/4 cup granola (optional)

Instructions:

Divide cottage cheese between two bowls.

Top with pineapple chunks and drizzle with honey.

Sprinkle with granola if desired.

Serve immediately.

Whole Wheat Banana Muffins

Servings: 12 muffins   **Calories:** 150 per muffin

Ingredients:

2 cups whole wheat flour

1 teaspoon baking soda

1/4 teaspoon salt

3 ripe bananas, mashed

1/2 cup honey

1/4 cup melted coconut oil

1 teaspoon vanilla extract

1 egg

Instructions:

Preheat the oven to 350°F (175°C) and line a muffin tin with paper liners.

In a large bowl, mix flour, baking soda, and salt.

In another bowl, combine mashed bananas, honey, melted coconut oil, vanilla extract, and egg.

Add the wet ingredients to the dry ingredients and mix until just combined.

Spoon the batter into the muffin tin, filling each cup about 3/4 full.

Bake for 18-20 minutes or until a toothpick inserted into the center comes out clean.

Cool on a wire rack and serve.

Chia Seed Pudding with Mango

Servings: 2   **Calories:** 200 per serving

Ingredients:

1/4 cup chia seeds

1 cup almond milk

1 tablespoon honey

1 ripe mango, diced

Instructions:

In a bowl, combine chia seeds, almond milk, and honey.

Stir well and refrigerate for at least 2 hours or overnight.

Stir again before serving and top with diced mango.

Buckwheat Pancakes

Servings: 4   **Calories:** 190 per serving

Ingredients:

1 cup buckwheat flour

1 tablespoon baking powder

1/4 teaspoon salt

1 egg

1 cup almond milk

2 tablespoons melted coconut oil

1 tablespoon honey

Instructions:

In a bowl, mix buckwheat flour, baking powder, and salt.

In another bowl, whisk together egg, almond milk, melted coconut oil, and honey.

Combine wet and dry ingredients, mixing until smooth.

Heat a skillet over medium heat and lightly oil it.

Pour batter onto the skillet, forming pancakes.

Cook until bubbles form on the surface, then flip and cook until golden.

Serve with fresh fruit or syrup.

Ricotta and Berry Toast

Servings: 2   **Calories:** 200 per serving

Ingredients:

2 slices whole grain bread

1/2 cup ricotta cheese

1/2 cup mixed berries (blueberries, strawberries, raspberries)

1 tablespoon honey

Instructions:

Toast the whole grain bread.

Spread ricotta cheese on each slice.

Top with mixed berries.

Drizzle with honey and serve immediately.

Sweet Potato and Avocado Hash

Servings: 2   **Calories:** 210 per serving

Ingredients:

2 medium sweet potatoes, peeled and diced

1 avocado, diced

1 tablespoon olive oil

Salt and pepper to taste

Instructions:

Heat olive oil in a skillet over medium heat.

Add diced sweet potatoes and cook until tender and crispy, about 10-15 minutes.

Season with salt and pepper.

Remove from heat and stir in diced avocado.

Serve immediately.

Berry Chia Smoothie Bowl

Servings: 2   **Calories:** 180 per serving

Ingredients:

1 cup mixed berries (blueberries, strawberries, raspberries)

1 banana

1/2 cup almond milk

2 tablespoons chia seeds

1 tablespoon honey

1/4 cup granola (optional)

Instructions:

Blend mixed berries, banana, almond milk, chia seeds, and honey until smooth.

Pour into bowls.

Top with granola if desired.

Serve immediately.

Pumpkin Spice Overnight Oats

Servings: 2   **Calories:** 230 per serving

Ingredients:

1 cup rolled oats

1 cup almond milk

1/2 cup pumpkin puree

1 tablespoon honey

1 teaspoon pumpkin spice

Instructions:

In a jar or container, combine oats, almond milk, pumpkin puree, honey, and pumpkin spice.

Mix well, cover, and refrigerate overnight.

In the morning, stir and serve cold or warmed up.

3. LUNCH RECIPES

Healing Chicken Broth

Servings: 4   **Calories:** 150 per serving

Ingredients:

1 whole chicken, cut into pieces

10 cups water

2 carrots, chopped

2 celery stalks, chopped

1 onion, chopped

3 cloves garlic, crushed

1 tablespoon apple cider vinegar

1 bay leaf

Salt and pepper to taste

Instructions:

In a large pot, combine all ingredients.

Bring to a boil, then reduce heat and simmer for 3-4 hours.

Strain the broth and discard solids.

Serve warm.

Creamy Carrot Soup

Servings: 4   **Calories:** 160 per serving

Ingredients:

6 large carrots, peeled and chopped

1 onion, chopped

3 cups vegetable broth

1 cup coconut milk

1 tablespoon olive oil

Salt and pepper to taste

Instructions:

In a pot, heat olive oil over medium heat.

Add onion and carrots, sautéing until soft.

Add vegetable broth and bring to a boil.

Reduce heat and simmer until carrots are tender, about 20 minutes.

Puree the soup using an immersion blender or regular blender.

Stir in coconut milk, season with salt and pepper, and serve warm.

Lentil and Vegetable Stew

Servings: 4   **Calories:** 220 per serving

Ingredients:

1 cup lentils, rinsed

1 onion, chopped

2 carrots, chopped

2 celery stalks, chopped

4 cups vegetable broth

1 can diced tomatoes (14.5 oz)

2 cloves garlic, minced

1 teaspoon thyme

Salt and pepper to taste

Instructions:

In a pot, sauté onion, carrots, celery, and garlic until soft.

Add lentils, vegetable broth, diced tomatoes, thyme, salt, and pepper.

Bring to a boil, then reduce heat and simmer for 30 minutes or until lentils are tender.

Serve warm.

Quinoa and Veggie Salad

Servings: 4   **Calories:** 180 per serving

Ingredients:

1 cup quinoa, rinsed

2 cups water

1 cucumber, diced

1 bell pepper, diced

1 cup cherry tomatoes, halved

1/4 cup red onion, finely chopped

2 tablespoons olive oil

1 tablespoon lemon juice

Salt and pepper to taste

Instructions:

Cook quinoa in water according to package instructions.

In a large bowl, combine cooked quinoa, cucumber, bell pepper, cherry tomatoes, and red onion.

In a small bowl, whisk together olive oil, lemon juice, salt, and pepper.

Pour dressing over salad and toss to combine.

Serve chilled.

Spinach and Strawberry Salad

Servings: 4   **Calories:** 170 per serving

Ingredients:

6 cups fresh spinach

2 cups strawberries, sliced

1/4 cup almonds, sliced

1/4 cup feta cheese, crumbled

2 tablespoons balsamic vinegar

2 tablespoons olive oil

Salt and pepper to taste

Instructions:

In a large bowl, combine spinach, strawberries, almonds, and feta cheese.

In a small bowl, whisk together balsamic vinegar, olive oil, salt, and pepper.

Pour dressing over salad and toss to combine.

Serve immediately.

Chickpea and Avocado Salad

Servings: 4   **Calories:** 200 per serving

Ingredients:

1 can chickpeas (15 oz), drained and rinsed

1 avocado, diced

1 cucumber, diced

1/4 cup red onion, finely chopped

2 tablespoons lemon juice

2 tablespoons olive oil

Salt and pepper to taste

Instructions:

In a large bowl, combine chickpeas, avocado, cucumber, and red onion.

In a small bowl, whisk together lemon juice, olive oil, salt, and pepper.

Pour dressing over salad and toss to combine.

Serve immediately.

Turkey and Avocado Wrap

Servings: 2   **Calories:** 250 per serving

Ingredients:

2 whole wheat tortillas

4 slices turkey breast

1 avocado, sliced

1 cup mixed greens

1/4 cup hummus

Instructions:

Spread hummus evenly on each tortilla.

Layer turkey slices, avocado, and mixed greens on top.

Roll up the tortillas tightly and slice in half.

Serve immediately.

Grilled Vegetable Sandwich

Servings: 2   **Calories:** 230 per serving

Ingredients:

1 zucchini, sliced

1 eggplant, sliced

1 red bell pepper, sliced

1 yellow bell pepper, sliced

4 slices whole grain bread

2 tablespoons olive oil

2 tablespoons pesto

Salt and pepper to taste

Instructions:

Preheat grill or grill pan over medium heat.

Brush vegetables with olive oil and season with salt and pepper.

Grill vegetables until tender and slightly charred.

Spread pesto on each slice of bread.

Layer grilled vegetables on two slices of bread and top with the remaining slices.

Serve immediately.

Tuna Salad on Whole Grain Bread

Servings: 2   **Calories:** 210 per serving

Ingredients:

1 can tuna (5 oz), drained

1/4 cup Greek yogurt

1 tablespoon lemon juice

1 celery stalk, finely chopped

Salt and pepper to taste

4 slices whole grain bread

1 cup mixed greens

Instructions:

In a bowl, combine tuna, Greek yogurt, lemon juice, celery, salt, and pepper.

Mix well until combined.

Spread tuna salad on two slices of bread.

Top with mixed greens and the remaining slices of bread.

Serve immediately.

Baked Salmon with Steamed Asparagus

Servings: 2   **Calories:** 250 per serving

Ingredients:

2 salmon fillets

1 bunch asparagus, trimmed

1 lemon, sliced

1 tablespoon olive oil

Salt and pepper to taste

Instructions:

Preheat oven to 375°F (190°C).

Place salmon fillets on a baking sheet lined with parchment paper.

Drizzle with olive oil and season with salt and pepper.

Top each fillet with lemon slices.

Bake for 15-20 minutes or until salmon is cooked through.

Meanwhile, steam asparagus until tender, about 5-7 minutes.

Serve salmon with steamed asparagus.

Broccoli and Cheddar Soup

Servings: 4   **Calories:** 200 per serving

Ingredients:

2 cups broccoli florets

1 onion, chopped

2 cups vegetable broth

1 cup milk

1 cup shredded cheddar cheese

2 tablespoons butter

2 tablespoons all-purpose flour

Salt and pepper to taste

Instructions:

In a pot, melt butter over medium heat.

Add onion and cook until soft.

Stir in flour and cook for 1 minute.

Gradually add vegetable broth, stirring constantly.

Add broccoli and bring to a boil.

Reduce heat and simmer until broccoli is tender, about 10 minutes.

Use an immersion blender to puree the soup until smooth.

Stir in milk and cheddar cheese, cooking until cheese is melted.

Season with salt and pepper, and serve warm.

Chicken and Rice Casserole

Servings: 4   **Calories:** 300 per serving

Ingredients:

2 cups cooked brown rice

2 cups cooked chicken, shredded

1 cup frozen peas and carrots

1 cup low-sodium chicken broth

1/2 cup Greek yogurt

1/2 cup shredded mozzarella cheese

Salt and pepper to taste

Instructions:

Preheat oven to 350°F (175°C).

In a large bowl, combine cooked rice, chicken, peas and carrots, chicken broth, and Greek yogurt.

Season with salt and pepper.

Transfer mixture to a baking dish.

Sprinkle shredded mozzarella cheese on top.

Bake for 20-25 minutes, or until heated through and cheese is melted.

Serve warm.

Turkey and Vegetable Stir-Fry

Servings: 4   **Calories:** 220 per serving

Ingredients:

1 pound ground turkey

1 bell pepper, sliced

1 zucchini, sliced

1 carrot, julienned

1 cup snap peas

2 tablespoons soy sauce

1 tablespoon olive oil

1 teaspoon ginger, minced

2 cloves garlic, minced

Salt and pepper to taste

Instructions:

Heat olive oil in a large skillet over medium heat.

Add ground turkey, cooking until browned.

Add ginger and garlic, cooking until fragrant.

Add bell pepper, zucchini, carrot, and snap peas.

Stir-fry until vegetables are tender-crisp.

Stir in soy sauce, and season with salt and pepper.

Serve immediately.

Quinoa Stuffed Bell Peppers

Servings: 4   **Calories:** 250 per serving

Ingredients:

4 bell peppers, tops cut off and seeds removed

1 cup cooked quinoa

1 can black beans (15 oz), drained and rinsed

1 cup corn kernels

1 cup diced tomatoes

1 teaspoon cumin

1/2 cup shredded cheddar cheese

Salt and pepper to taste

Instructions:

Preheat oven to 375°F (190°C).

In a bowl, combine cooked quinoa, black beans, corn, diced tomatoes, cumin, salt, and pepper.

Stuff each bell pepper with the quinoa mixture.

Place stuffed bell peppers in a baking dish.

Sprinkle shredded cheddar cheese on top.

Cover with foil and bake for 25-30 minutes.

Remove foil and bake for an additional 10 minutes, until cheese is melted.

Serve warm.

Vegetable and Hummus Wrap

Servings: 2   **Calories:** 180 per serving

Ingredients:

2 whole wheat tortillas

1 cup mixed greens

1/2 cucumber, sliced

1/2 bell pepper, sliced

1/4 cup shredded carrots

1/2 cup hummus

Instructions:

Spread hummus evenly on each tortilla.

Layer mixed greens, cucumber, bell pepper, and shredded carrots on top.

Roll up the tortillas tightly and slice in half.

Serve immediately.

Spinach and Feta Stuffed Chicken Breast

Servings: 2   **Calories:** 260 per serving

Ingredients:

2 boneless, skinless chicken breasts

1 cup fresh spinach, chopped

1/4 cup feta cheese, crumbled

1 tablespoon olive oil

Salt and pepper to taste

Instructions:

Preheat oven to 375°F (190°C).

Using a sharp knife, cut a pocket into each chicken breast.

In a bowl, combine chopped spinach and feta cheese.

Stuff the chicken breasts with the spinach and feta mixture.

Secure with toothpicks if needed.

Season with salt and pepper.

Heat olive oil in an oven-safe skillet over medium heat.

Brown chicken breasts on both sides, about 3-4 minutes per side.

Transfer skillet to the oven and bake for 20-25 minutes, until chicken is cooked through.

Serve warm.

Butternut Squash and Lentil Salad

Servings: 4   **Calories:** 220 per serving

Ingredients:

1 butternut squash, peeled and cubed

1 cup cooked lentils

1/4 cup red onion, finely chopped

2 cups mixed greens

2 tablespoons olive oil

1 tablespoon balsamic vinegar

Salt and pepper to taste

Instructions:

Preheat oven to 400°F (200°C).

Toss butternut squash cubes with 1 tablespoon olive oil, salt, and pepper.

Spread on a baking sheet and roast for 25-30 minutes, until tender and lightly browned.

In a large bowl, combine roasted butternut squash, cooked lentils, red onion, and mixed greens.

In a small bowl, whisk together the remaining olive oil and balsamic vinegar.

Pour dressing over the salad and toss to combine.

Serve immediately.

Tomato Basil Soup

Servings: 4   **Calories:** 180 per serving

Ingredients:

4 cups diced tomatoes

1 onion, chopped

2 cloves garlic, minced

2 cups vegetable broth

1/2 cup fresh basil, chopped

1 tablespoon olive oil

Salt and pepper to taste

Instructions:

In a pot, heat olive oil over medium heat.

Add onion and garlic, cooking until soft.

Add diced tomatoes and vegetable broth.

Bring to a boil, then reduce heat and simmer for 20 minutes.

Use an immersion blender to puree the soup until smooth.

Stir in fresh basil, season with salt and pepper, and serve warm.

Greek Salad with Grilled Chicken

Servings: 2   **Calories:** 250 per serving

Ingredients:

2 boneless, skinless chicken breasts

4 cups mixed greens

1/2 cucumber, sliced

1/2 cup cherry tomatoes, halved

1/4 cup red onion, sliced

1/4 cup feta cheese, crumbled

2 tablespoons olive oil

1 tablespoon lemon juice

1 teaspoon oregano

Salt and pepper to taste

Instructions:

Season chicken breasts with salt, pepper, and oregano.

Grill chicken until cooked through, about 6-8 minutes per side.

In a large bowl, combine mixed greens, cucumber, cherry tomatoes, red onion, and feta cheese.

In a small bowl, whisk together olive oil and lemon juice.

Pour dressing over salad and toss to combine.

Slice grilled chicken and place on top of the salad.

Serve immediately.

Sweet Potato and Black Bean Tacos

Servings: 4   **Calories:** 230 per serving

Ingredients:

2 large sweet potatoes, peeled and diced

1 can black beans (15 oz), drained and rinsed

8 small corn tortillas

1/2 cup salsa

1/4 cup cilantro, chopped

2 tablespoons olive oil

1 teaspoon cumin

Salt and pepper to taste

Instructions:

Preheat oven to 400°F (200°C).

Toss sweet potato cubes with olive oil, cumin, salt, and pepper.

Spread on a baking sheet and roast for 25-30 minutes, until tender.

Warm corn tortillas in a dry skillet over medium heat.

In a bowl, combine roasted sweet potatoes and black beans.

Fill each tortilla with the sweet potato and black bean mixture.

Top with salsa and chopped cilantro.

Serve immediately.

4. DINNER RECIPES

Baked Cod with Lemon and Dill

Servings: 4   **Calories:** 180 per serving

Ingredients:

4 cod fillets

2 lemons, sliced

2 tablespoons olive oil

2 tablespoons fresh dill, chopped

Salt and pepper to taste

Instructions:

Preheat oven to 375°F (190°C).

Place cod fillets on a baking sheet lined with parchment paper.

Drizzle with olive oil and season with salt and pepper.

Top each fillet with lemon slices and sprinkle with fresh dill.

Bake for 15-20 minutes, until the fish is opaque and flakes easily with a fork.

Serve warm.

Chicken and Vegetable Skewers

Servings: 4   **Calories:** 220 per serving

Ingredients:

1 pound chicken breast, cubed

1 red bell pepper, cubed

1 yellow bell pepper, cubed

1 zucchini, sliced

1 red onion, cubed

2 tablespoons olive oil

2 tablespoons lemon juice

1 teaspoon dried oregano

Salt and pepper to taste

Instructions:

Preheat grill to medium-high heat.

In a bowl, combine olive oil, lemon juice, oregano, salt, and pepper.

Thread chicken and vegetables onto skewers.

Brush with the olive oil mixture.

Grill for 10-12 minutes, turning occasionally, until chicken is cooked through and vegetables are tender.

Serve warm.

Turkey Meatballs with Zucchini Noodles

Servings: 4   **Calories:** 250 per serving

Ingredients:

1 pound ground turkey

1/4 cup breadcrumbs

1/4 cup grated Parmesan cheese

1 egg

2 cloves garlic, minced

2 tablespoons fresh parsley, chopped

Salt and pepper to taste

4 zucchinis, spiralized into noodles

2 tablespoons olive oil

Instructions:

Preheat oven to 375°F (190°C).

In a bowl, combine ground turkey, breadcrumbs, Parmesan cheese, egg, garlic, parsley, salt, and pepper.

Form into meatballs and place on a baking sheet lined with parchment paper.

Bake for 20-25 minutes, until meatballs are cooked through.

In a large skillet, heat olive oil over medium heat.

Add zucchini noodles and sauté for 2-3 minutes, until tender.

Serve meatballs over zucchini noodles.

Salmon with Quinoa and Asparagus

Servings: 4   **Calories:** 270 per serving

Ingredients:

4 salmon fillets

1 cup quinoa, rinsed

2 cups water

1 bunch asparagus, trimmed

2 tablespoons olive oil

1 lemon, juiced

Salt and pepper to taste

Instructions:

Preheat oven to 375°F (190°C).

Place salmon fillets on a baking sheet lined with parchment paper.

Drizzle with olive oil, lemon juice, salt, and pepper.

Bake for 15-20 minutes, until salmon is cooked through.

Meanwhile, bring water to a boil in a pot.

Add quinoa, reduce heat, cover, and simmer for 15 minutes, until water is absorbed.

Steam asparagus until tender, about 5-7 minutes.

Serve salmon with quinoa and asparagus.

Vegetable Stir-Fry with Tofu

Servings: 4   **Calories:** 200 per serving

Ingredients:

1 block firm tofu, cubed

1 bell pepper, sliced

1 zucchini, sliced

1 cup snap peas

1 carrot, julienned

2 tablespoons soy sauce

1 tablespoon olive oil

1 teaspoon ginger, minced

2 cloves garlic, minced

Salt and pepper to taste

Instructions:

Heat olive oil in a large skillet over medium heat.

Add tofu cubes and cook until browned on all sides.

Remove tofu from skillet and set aside.

Add ginger and garlic to the skillet, cooking until fragrant.

Add bell pepper, zucchini, snap peas, and carrot.

Stir-fry until vegetables are tender-crisp.

Return tofu to the skillet and stir in soy sauce.

Season with salt and pepper.

Serve warm.

Baked Eggplant Parmesan

Servings: 4   **Calories:** 240 per serving

Ingredients:

2 eggplants, sliced into rounds

1 cup marinara sauce

1 cup shredded mozzarella cheese

1/4 cup grated Parmesan cheese

1 cup breadcrumbs

2 eggs, beaten

2 tablespoons olive oil

Salt and pepper to taste

Instructions:

Preheat oven to 375°F (190°C).

Dip eggplant slices in beaten eggs, then coat with breadcrumbs.

Heat olive oil in a large skillet over medium heat.

Cook eggplant slices until golden brown on both sides.

In a baking dish, layer half of the eggplant slices, marinara sauce, mozzarella cheese, and Parmesan cheese.

Repeat the layers with the remaining ingredients.

Bake for 20-25 minutes, until cheese is melted and bubbly.

Serve warm.

Shrimp and Vegetable Skillet

Servings: 4   **Calories:** 210 per serving

Ingredients:

1 pound shrimp, peeled and deveined

1 bell pepper, sliced

1 zucchini, sliced

1 cup cherry tomatoes, halved

2 tablespoons olive oil

2 cloves garlic, minced

1 teaspoon paprika

Salt and pepper to taste

Instructions:

Heat olive oil in a large skillet over medium heat.

Add garlic and cook until fragrant.

Add shrimp, bell pepper, zucchini, and cherry tomatoes.

Sprinkle with paprika, salt, and pepper.

Cook until shrimp is pink and vegetables are tender, about 5-7 minutes.

Serve warm.

Turkey and Spinach Stuffed Peppers

Servings: 4   **Calories:** 230 per serving

Ingredients:

4 bell peppers, tops cut off and seeds removed

1 pound ground turkey

2 cups fresh spinach, chopped

1/2 cup quinoa, cooked

1/2 cup tomato sauce

1 onion, chopped

2 cloves garlic, minced

2 tablespoons olive oil

Salt and pepper to taste

Instructions:

Preheat oven to 375°F (190°C).

Heat olive oil in a large skillet over medium heat. Add onion and garlic, cooking until soft. Add ground turkey, cooking until browned.

Stir in chopped spinach and cook until wilted. Add cooked quinoa and tomato sauce, stirring to combine. Season with salt and pepper.

Stuff each bell pepper with the turkey mixture. Place stuffed peppers in a baking dish. Cover with foil and bake for 25-30 minutes.

Serve warm.

Baked Lemon Herb Chicken

Servings: 4   **Calories:** 210 per serving

Ingredients:

4 boneless, skinless chicken breasts

2 lemons, sliced

2 tablespoons olive oil

2 tablespoons fresh rosemary, chopped

2 cloves garlic, minced

Salt and pepper to taste

Instructions:

Preheat oven to 375°F (190°C).

Place chicken breasts in a baking dish.

Drizzle with olive oil and season with salt, pepper, garlic, and rosemary.

Top each chicken breast with lemon slices.

Bake for 25-30 minutes, until chicken is cooked through.

Serve warm.

Veggie-Packed Pasta Primavera

Servings: 4   **Calories:** 230 per serving

Ingredients:

8 ounces whole wheat pasta

1 cup broccoli florets

1 bell pepper, sliced

1 zucchini, sliced

1 cup cherry tomatoes, halved

1/4 cup grated Parmesan cheese

2 tablespoons olive oil

2 cloves garlic, minced

Salt and pepper to taste

Instructions:

Cook pasta according to package instructions. Drain and set aside.

Heat olive oil in a large skillet over medium heat.

Add garlic and cook until fragrant.

Add broccoli, bell pepper, zucchini, and cherry tomatoes.

Cook until vegetables are tender, about 5-7 minutes.

Add cooked pasta to the skillet, stirring to combine.

Season with salt and pepper.

Sprinkle with Parmesan cheese and serve warm.

Lemon Garlic Baked Tilapia

Servings: 4   **Calories:** 180 per serving

Ingredients:

4 tilapia fillets

3 tablespoons lemon juice

2 cloves garlic, minced

1 tablespoon olive oil

1 teaspoon dried basil

1 teaspoon dried parsley

Salt and pepper to taste

Instructions:

Preheat oven to 375°F (190°C).

Place tilapia fillets in a baking dish.

In a small bowl, mix lemon juice, garlic, olive oil, basil, parsley, salt, and pepper.

Pour mixture over the tilapia fillets.

Bake for 20-25 minutes, until fish is flaky and cooked through.

Serve warm with a side of steamed vegetables.

Chicken and Rice Stuffed Zucchini

Servings: 4   **Calories:** 220 per serving

Ingredients:

4 medium zucchinis

1 cup cooked brown rice

1 cup cooked chicken, shredded

1/2 cup marinara sauce

1/4 cup grated Parmesan cheese

1 onion, finely chopped

2 cloves garlic, minced

2 tablespoons olive oil

Salt and pepper to taste

Instructions:

Preheat oven to 375°F (190°C).

Cut zucchinis in half lengthwise and scoop out the centers.

In a skillet, heat olive oil over medium heat. Add onion and garlic, cooking until soft.

Add shredded chicken, cooked rice, and marinara sauce, stirring to combine. Season with salt and pepper.

Fill zucchini halves with the chicken and rice mixture. Place stuffed zucchinis in a baking dish. Sprinkle with grated Parmesan cheese. Bake for 25-30 minutes, until zucchinis are tender.

Serve warm.

Herb-Roasted Chicken Thighs

Servings: 4   **Calories:** 250 per serving

Ingredients:

8 chicken thighs, bone-in and skin-on

2 tablespoons olive oil

1 tablespoon dried rosemary

1 tablespoon dried thyme

1 lemon, sliced

3 cloves garlic, minced

Salt and pepper to taste

Instructions:

Preheat oven to 375°F (190°C).

In a large bowl, mix olive oil, rosemary, thyme, garlic, salt, and pepper.

Add chicken thighs and toss to coat evenly.

Place chicken thighs on a baking sheet.

Top with lemon slices.

Roast for 35-40 minutes, until chicken is cooked through and skin is crispy.

Serve warm.

Lentil and Sweet Potato Curry

Servings: 4   **Calories:** 240 per serving

Ingredients:

1 cup lentils, rinsed

2 medium sweet potatoes, peeled and cubed

1 onion, chopped

3 cloves garlic, minced

1 can coconut milk (14 oz)

2 cups vegetable broth

1 tablespoon curry powder

1 teaspoon turmeric

2 tablespoons olive oil

Salt and pepper to taste

Instructions:

In a large pot, heat olive oil over medium heat. Add onion and garlic, cooking until soft. Stir in curry powder and turmeric, cooking for 1 minute. Add lentils, sweet potatoes, coconut milk, and vegetable broth.

Bring to a boil, then reduce heat and simmer for 25-30 minutes, until lentils and sweet potatoes are tender. Season with salt and pepper.

Serve warm.

Beef and Vegetable Stir-Fry

Servings: 4   **Calories:** 260 per serving

Ingredients:

1 pound beef sirloin, thinly sliced

1 bell pepper, sliced

1 broccoli head, cut into florets

1 carrot, julienned

1 onion, sliced

2 tablespoons soy sauce

2 tablespoons olive oil

1 teaspoon ginger, minced

2 cloves garlic, minced

Salt and pepper to taste

Instructions:

Heat olive oil in a large skillet over medium heat. Add ginger and garlic, cooking until fragrant. Add beef and cook until browned. Remove beef from skillet and set aside.

Add bell pepper, broccoli, carrot, and onion to the skillet. Stir-fry until vegetables are tender-crisp.

Return beef to the skillet and stir in soy sauce. Season with salt and pepper.

Serve warm.

Chicken and Broccoli Alfredo

Servings: 4   **Calories:** 280 per serving

Ingredients:

8 ounces whole wheat pasta

2 cups cooked chicken, shredded

1 broccoli head, cut into florets

1 cup Greek yogurt

1/2 cup grated Parmesan cheese

2 cloves garlic, minced

2 tablespoons olive oil

Salt and pepper to taste

Instructions:

Cook pasta according to package instructions. Drain and set aside.

Steam broccoli until tender, about 5-7 minutes.

In a large skillet, heat olive oil over medium heat. Add garlic and cook until fragrant.

Stir in Greek yogurt and Parmesan cheese, cooking until cheese is melted.

Add cooked chicken and steamed broccoli, stirring to combine. Season with salt and pepper. Toss pasta with the Alfredo sauce.

Serve warm.

Baked Falafel with Tahini Sauce

Servings: 4   **Calories:** 230 per servin

Ingredients:

1 can chickpeas (15 oz), drained and rinsed

1/4 cup fresh parsley, chopped

2 cloves garlic, minced

1 teaspoon cumin

1 teaspoon coriander

2 tablespoons olive oil

Salt and pepper to taste

1/2 cup tahini

1/4 cup lemon juice

1/4 cup water

Instructions:

Preheat oven to 375°F (190°C).

In a food processor, combine chickpeas, parsley, garlic, cumin, coriander, olive oil, salt, and pepper.

Pulse until mixture is well combined but still slightly chunky.

Form mixture into small patties and place on a baking sheet lined with parchment paper. Bake for 20-25 minutes, until golden brown.

In a small bowl, whisk together tahini, lemon juice, and water until smooth.

Serve falafel with tahini sauce.

Quinoa and Black Bean Stuffed Peppers

Servings: 4   **Calories:** 240 per serving

Ingredients:

4 bell peppers, tops cut off and seeds removed

1 cup cooked quinoa

1 can black beans (15 oz), drained and rinsed

1 cup corn kernels

1/2 cup salsa

1/4 cup shredded cheddar cheese

1 onion, finely chopped

2 cloves garlic, minced

2 tablespoons olive oil

Salt and pepper to taste

Instructions:

Preheat oven to 375°F (190°C).

In a large skillet, heat olive oil over medium heat. Add onion and garlic, cooking until soft. Stir in cooked quinoa, black beans, corn, and salsa, cooking until heated through. Season with salt and pepper.

Stuff each bell pepper with the quinoa mixture. Place stuffed peppers in a baking dish. Sprinkle with shredded cheddar cheese. Cover with foil and bake for 25-30 minutes.

Serve warm.

Herb-Crusted Pork Tenderloin

Servings: 4   **Calories:** 250 per serving

Ingredients:

1 pork tenderloin (1 pound)

2 tablespoons olive oil

2 tablespoons fresh rosemary, chopped

2 tablespoons fresh thyme, chopped

2 cloves garlic, minced

Salt and pepper to taste

Instructions:

Preheat oven to 375°F (190°C).

In a small bowl, combine olive oil, rosemary, thyme, garlic, salt, and pepper.

Rub mixture all over the pork tenderloin.

Place tenderloin in a baking dish.

Roast for 25-30 minutes, until the internal temperature reaches 145°F (63°C).

Let rest for 5 minutes before slicing.

Serve warm.

5. SNACKS AND SIDE DISHES

Hummus and Veggie Sticks

Servings: 4   **Calories:** 150 per serving

Ingredients:

1 can chickpeas (15 oz), drained and rinsed

1/4 cup tahini

2 tablespoons olive oil

2 tablespoons lemon juice

2 cloves garlic, minced

1/2 teaspoon cumin

Salt and pepper to taste

1 cucumber, sliced

2 carrots, cut into sticks

1 bell pepper, sliced

Instructions:

In a food processor, combine chickpeas, tahini, olive oil, lemon juice, garlic, cumin, salt, and pepper.

Blend until smooth and creamy.

Serve hummus with cucumber, carrot, and bell pepper sticks.

Baked Sweet Potato Fries

Servings: 4   **Calories:** 160 per serving

Ingredients:

2 large sweet potatoes, peeled and cut into fries

2 tablespoons olive oil

1 teaspoon paprika

1/2 teaspoon garlic powder

Salt and pepper to taste

Instructions:

Preheat oven to 425°F (220°C).

In a large bowl, toss sweet potato fries with olive oil, paprika, garlic powder, salt, and pepper.

Spread fries in a single layer on a baking sheet lined with parchment paper.

Bake for 25-30 minutes, turning halfway, until fries are crispy and golden brown.

Serve warm.

Cucumber and Avocado Salad

Servings: 4   **Calories:** 140 per serving

Ingredients:

2 cucumbers, sliced

2 avocados, diced

1/4 red onion, thinly sliced

2 tablespoons fresh dill, chopped

2 tablespoons olive oil

1 tablespoon lemon juice

Salt and pepper to taste

Instructions:

In a large bowl, combine cucumbers, avocados, red onion, and fresh dill.

In a small bowl, whisk together olive oil, lemon juice, salt, and pepper.

Pour dressing over the salad and toss to combine.

Serve immediately.

Quinoa Tabbouleh

Servings: 4   **Calories:** 180 per serving

Ingredients:

1 cup quinoa, rinsed and cooked

1 cup cherry tomatoes, halved

1 cucumber, diced

1/4 cup fresh parsley, chopped

1/4 cup fresh mint, chopped

1/4 cup lemon juice

2 tablespoons olive oil

Salt and pepper to taste

Instructions:

In a large bowl, combine cooked quinoa, cherry tomatoes, cucumber, parsley, and mint.

In a small bowl, whisk together lemon juice, olive oil, salt, and pepper.

Pour dressing over the quinoa mixture and toss to combine.

Serve chilled or at room temperature.

Apple Slices with Almond Butter

Servings: 4   **Calories:** 130 per serving

Ingredients:

2 large apples, sliced

1/2 cup almond butter

1 teaspoon cinnamon

Instructions:

Arrange apple slices on a serving plate.

Serve almond butter in a small bowl.

Sprinkle cinnamon over the apple slices.

Dip apple slices into almond butter and enjoy.

Steamed Asparagus with Lemon

Servings: 4   **Calories:** 60 per serving

Ingredients:

1 bunch asparagus, trimmed

1 tablespoon olive oil

1 lemon, juiced

Salt and pepper to taste

Instructions:

Steam asparagus until tender, about 5-7 minutes.

In a small bowl, whisk together olive oil, lemon juice, salt, and pepper.

Drizzle dressing over steamed asparagus.

Serve warm or chilled.

Roasted Chickpeas

Servings: 4   **Calories:** 130 per serving

Ingredients:

1 can chickpeas (15 oz), drained and rinsed

2 tablespoons olive oil

1 teaspoon paprika

1/2 teaspoon garlic powder

Salt and pepper to taste

Instructions:

Preheat oven to 400°F (200°C).

In a large bowl, toss chickpeas with olive oil, paprika, garlic powder, salt, and pepper.

Spread chickpeas in a single layer on a baking sheet lined with parchment paper.

Roast for 20-25 minutes, shaking the pan halfway through, until chickpeas are crispy.

Serve warm or at room temperature.

Baked Zucchini Chips

Servings: 4   **Calories:** 110 per serving

Ingredients:

2 zucchinis, thinly sliced

2 tablespoons olive oil

1/2 teaspoon garlic powder

1/2 teaspoon paprika

Salt and pepper to taste

Instructions:

Preheat oven to 425°F (220°C).

In a large bowl, toss zucchini slices with olive oil, garlic powder, paprika, salt, and pepper.

Arrange slices in a single layer on a baking sheet lined with parchment paper.

Bake for 15-20 minutes, turning halfway, until chips are golden and crispy.

Serve warm or at room temperature.

Cottage Cheese and Pineapple

Servings: 4   **Calories:** 100 per serving

Ingredients:

2 cups cottage cheese

1 cup pineapple chunks

1 tablespoon honey (optional)

Instructions:

Divide cottage cheese into four servings.

Top each serving with pineapple chunks.

Drizzle with honey if desired.

Serve immediately.

Spinach and Feta Stuffed Mushrooms

Servings: 4   **Calories:** 90 per serving

Ingredients:

16 large button mushrooms, stems removed

2 cups fresh spinach, chopped

1/2 cup feta cheese, crumbled

1/4 cup breadcrumbs

2 cloves garlic, minced

2 tablespoons olive oil

Salt and pepper to taste

Instructions:

Preheat oven to 375°F (190°C).

In a skillet, heat olive oil over medium heat. Add garlic and cook until fragrant. Add chopped spinach and cook until wilted.

Remove from heat and stir in feta cheese, breadcrumbs, salt, and pepper. Spoon the mixture into the mushroom caps. Place stuffed mushrooms on a baking sheet lined with parchment paper.

Bake for 15-20 minutes, until mushrooms are tender and tops are golden.

Serve warm.

Carrot and Ginger Soup

Servings: 4   **Calories:** 120 per serving

Ingredients:

1 pound carrots, peeled and chopped

1 onion, chopped

2 cloves garlic, minced

1 tablespoon fresh ginger, grated

4 cups vegetable broth

2 tablespoons olive oil

Salt and pepper to taste

Instructions:

In a large pot, heat olive oil over medium heat.

Add onion, garlic, and ginger, cooking until soft.

Add chopped carrots and vegetable broth.

Bring to a boil, then reduce heat and simmer for 20-25 minutes, until carrots are tender.

Using an immersion blender, puree the soup until smooth.

Season with salt and pepper.

Serve warm.

Guacamole with Baked Pita Chips

Servings: 4   **Calories:** 180 per serving

Ingredients:

2 avocados, mashed

1/2 red onion, finely chopped

1 tomato, diced

1 lime, juiced

2 cloves garlic, minced

2 tablespoons fresh cilantro, chopped

Salt and pepper to taste

4 whole wheat pita breads, cut into wedges

2 tablespoons olive oil

Instructions:

Preheat oven to 375°F (190°C).

In a bowl, combine mashed avocados, red onion, tomato, lime juice, garlic, cilantro, salt, and pepper.

Place pita wedges on a baking sheet lined with parchment paper.

Brush with olive oil and sprinkle with a little salt.

Bake for 10-12 minutes, until crispy.

Serve guacamole with baked pita chips.

Apple and Cheddar Slices

Servings: 4   **Calories:** 150 per serving

Ingredients:

2 large apples, sliced

4 ounces cheddar cheese, sliced

Instructions:

Arrange apple slices on a serving plate.

Place a slice of cheddar cheese on each apple slice.

Serve immediately.

Roasted Cauliflower

Servings: 4   **Calories:** 100 per serving

Ingredients:

1 large head cauliflower, cut into florets

2 tablespoons olive oil

1 teaspoon paprika

1/2 teaspoon garlic powder

Salt and pepper to taste

Instructions:

Preheat oven to 400°F (200°C).

In a large bowl, toss cauliflower florets with olive oil, paprika, garlic powder, salt, and pepper.

Spread florets in a single layer on a baking sheet lined with parchment paper.

Roast for 25-30 minutes, turning halfway, until golden and tender.

Serve warm.

Tomato and Mozzarella Salad

Servings: 4   **Calories:** 130 per serving

Ingredients:

4 large tomatoes, sliced

8 ounces fresh mozzarella, sliced

1/4 cup fresh basil leaves

2 tablespoons olive oil

1 tablespoon balsamic vinegar

Salt and pepper to taste

Instructions:

Arrange tomato and mozzarella slices on a serving plate, alternating them.

Scatter fresh basil leaves on top.

Drizzle with olive oil and balsamic vinegar.

Season with salt and pepper.

Serve immediately.

Greek Yogurt and Cucumber Dip

Servings: 4   **Calories:** 80 per serving

Ingredients:

1 cup Greek yogurt

1 cucumber, grated and excess water squeezed out

2 cloves garlic, minced

2 tablespoons fresh dill, chopped

1 tablespoon lemon juice

Salt and pepper to taste

Instructions:

In a bowl, combine Greek yogurt, grated cucumber, garlic, dill, lemon juice, salt, and pepper.

Mix well and refrigerate for at least 30 minutes to allow flavors to meld.

Serve with vegetable sticks or pita bread.

Steamed Green Beans with Almonds

Servings: 4   **Calories:** 90 per serving

Ingredients:

1-pound green beans, trimmed

1/4 cup sliced almonds, toasted

2 tablespoons olive oil

1 lemon, zested

Salt and pepper to taste

Instructions:

Steam green beans until tender, about 5-7 minutes.

In a large bowl, toss green beans with olive oil, lemon zest, salt, and pepper.

Sprinkle with toasted almonds.

Serve warm.

Berry and Spinach Smoothie

Servings: 4   **Calories:** 110 per serving

Ingredients:

2 cups fresh spinach

1 cup mixed berries (strawberries, blueberries, raspberries)

1 banana

1 cup almond milk

1 tablespoon honey (optional)

Instructions:

In a blender, combine spinach, mixed berries, banana, almond milk, and honey.

Blend until smooth.

Serve immediately.

Roasted Bell Pepper and Hummus Wrap

Servings: 4   **Calories:** 180 per serving

Ingredients:

2 large bell peppers, roasted and sliced

1 cup hummus

4 whole wheat tortillas

1/2 cup fresh spinach leaves

1/4 cup feta cheese, crumbled

Instructions:

Spread hummus evenly over each tortilla.

Top with roasted bell pepper slices, spinach leaves, and crumbled feta cheese.

Roll up tortillas and cut in half.

Serve immediately.

6. DESSERTS AND SWEETS

Banana Ice Cream

Servings: 2   **Calories:** 120 per serving

Ingredients:

2 ripe bananas, sliced and frozen

1 teaspoon vanilla extract

1 tablespoon almond milk (optional)

Instructions:

Place frozen banana slices in a food processor.

Blend until smooth and creamy.

Add vanilla extract and blend again.

If needed, add almond milk for a smoother texture.

Serve immediately.

Chia Pudding with Berries

Servings: 4   **Calories:** 180 per serving

Ingredients:

1/2 cup chia seeds

2 cups almond milk

1 teaspoon vanilla extract

2 tablespoons honey

1 cup mixed berries

Instructions:

In a bowl, combine chia seeds, almond milk, vanilla extract, and honey.

Stir well and let sit for 5 minutes.

Stir again to prevent clumping.

Cover and refrigerate for at least 2 hours or overnight.

Serve with mixed berries on top.

Mango Sorbet

Servings: 4   Calories: 110 per serving

Ingredients:

3 ripe mangoes, peeled and chopped

1/4 cup honey

1 tablespoon lime juice

Instructions:

Place chopped mangoes in a blender. Add honey and lime juice. Blend until smooth.

Pour mixture into a shallow container.

Freeze for at least 4 hours, stirring every hour to break up ice crystals.

Serve.

Baked Pears with Honey and Ginger

Servings: 4   **Calories:** 140 per serving

Ingredients:

4 ripe pears, halved and cored

2 tablespoons honey

1 teaspoon ground ginger

Instructions:

Preheat the oven to 350°F (175°C).

Place pear halves in a baking dish.

Drizzle with honey and sprinkle with ginger.

Bake for 20-25 minutes until tender.

Serve warm.

Rice Pudding

Servings: 4   **Calories:** 220 per serving

Ingredients:

1/2 cup short-grain rice

2 cups almond milk

1/4 cup honey

1 teaspoon vanilla extract

1/2 teaspoon ground cinnamon

Instructions:

In a saucepan, combine rice and almond milk.

Bring to a boil, then reduce heat to low.

Simmer, stirring frequently, for 20-25 minutes until rice is tender.

Stir in honey, vanilla extract, and cinnamon.

Serve warm or chilled.

Coconut Macaroons

Servings: 12   **Calories:** 100 per serving

Ingredients:

2 cups shredded coconut

2 egg whites

1/4 cup honey

1 teaspoon vanilla extract

Instructions:

Preheat the oven to 325°F (165°C).

In a bowl, mix shredded coconut, egg whites, honey, and vanilla extract.

Drop spoonfuls of the mixture onto a baking sheet lined with parchment paper.

Bake for 15-20 minutes until golden brown.

Cool on a wire rack.

Blueberry Muffins

Servings: 12   **Calories:** 150 per serving

Ingredients:

1 1/2 cups whole wheat flour

1/2 cup almond flour

1/4 cup honey

1 tablespoon baking powder

1/2 teaspoon salt

1 cup almond milk

1/4 cup coconut oil, melted

2 eggs

1 cup fresh blueberries

Instructions:

Preheat the oven to 375°F (190°C).

In a bowl, combine flours, baking powder, and salt.

In another bowl, whisk almond milk, coconut oil, honey, and eggs.

Add wet ingredients to dry ingredients and mix until just combined. Fold in blueberries. Divide batter into a muffin tin lined with paper cups.

Bake for 20-25 minutes until a toothpick inserted into the center comes out clean.

Cool on a wire rack.

Pumpkin Smoothie

Servings: 2   **Calories:** 180 per serving

Ingredients:

1 cup pumpkin puree

1 banana

1 cup almond milk

1 tablespoon honey

1/2 teaspoon ground cinnamon

1/4 teaspoon ground nutmeg

Instructions:

Place all ingredients in a blender.

Blend until smooth.

Pour into glasses and serve immediately.

Applesauce Muffins

Servings: 12   **Calories:** 140 per serving

Ingredients:

1 1/2 cups whole wheat flour

1/2 cup rolled oats

1/2 cup applesauce

1/4 cup honey

1/2 cup almond milk

1/4 cup coconut oil, melted

1 teaspoon baking powder

1/2 teaspoon baking soda

1/2 teaspoon ground cinnamon

1/4 teaspoon salt

2 eggs

Instructions:

Preheat the oven to 350°F (175°C).

In a bowl, mix flour, oats, baking powder, baking soda, cinnamon, and salt.

In another bowl, whisk applesauce, honey, almond milk, coconut oil, and eggs.

Combine wet and dry ingredients until just mixed.

Divide batter into a muffin tin lined with paper cups.

Bake for 20-25 minutes until a toothpick inserted comes out clean.

Cool on a wire rack.

Strawberry Chia Jam

Servings: 10   **Calories:** 40 per serving

Ingredients:

2 cups fresh strawberries, hulled and chopped

2 tablespoons honey

2 tablespoons chia seeds

1 teaspoon lemon juice

Instructions:

In a saucepan, cook strawberries over medium heat until they start to break down.

Mash the strawberries with a fork or potato masher.

Stir in honey and lemon juice.

Remove from heat and stir in chia seeds.

Let cool and thicken for 1 hour.

Store in the refrigerator.

Banana Oat Cookies

Servings: 12   **Calories:** 90 per serving

Ingredients:

2 ripe bananas, mashed

1 cup rolled oats

1/4 cup almond butter

1 teaspoon vanilla extract

Instructions:

Preheat the oven to 350°F (175°C).

In a bowl, mix mashed bananas, oats, almond butter, and vanilla extract.

Drop spoonfuls of the mixture onto a baking sheet lined with parchment paper.

Flatten slightly with a fork.

Bake for 12-15 minutes until golden brown.

Cool on a wire rack.

Almond Flour Brownies

Servings: 16   **Calories:** 130 per serving

Ingredients:

1 1/2 cups almond flour

1/4 cup cocoa powder

1/4 cup honey

1/4 cup coconut oil, melted

2 eggs

1 teaspoon vanilla extract

1/2 teaspoon baking soda

1/4 teaspoon salt

Instructions:

Preheat the oven to 350°F (175°C).

In a bowl, mix almond flour, cocoa powder, baking soda, and salt.

In another bowl, whisk honey, coconut oil, eggs, and vanilla extract.

Combine wet and dry ingredients until smooth.

Pour batter into a greased 8x8-inch baking dish.

Bake for 20-25 minutes until a toothpick inserted comes out clean.

Cool before cutting into squares.

Avocado Chocolate Mousse

Servings: 4   Calories: 180 per serving

Ingredients:

2 ripe avocados

1/4 cup cocoa powder

1/4 cup honey

1 teaspoon vanilla extract

Pinch of salt

Instructions:

In a blender, combine avocados, cocoa powder, honey, vanilla extract, and salt.

Blend until smooth and creamy.

Refrigerate for at least 1 hour before serving.

Peach Frozen Yogurt

Servings: 4   **Calories:** 120 per serving

Ingredients:

3 cups frozen peaches

1 cup Greek yogurt

1/4 cup honey

1 teaspoon lemon juice

Instructions:

In a blender, combine peaches, Greek yogurt, honey, and lemon juice.

Blend until smooth.

Serve immediately or freeze for a firmer texture.

Lemon Blueberry Bars

Servings: 12   **Calories:** 140 per serving

Ingredients:

1 1/2 cups almond flour

1/4 cup coconut oil, melted

1/4 cup honey

1 teaspoon vanilla extract

1 cup fresh blueberries

Zest and juice of 1 lemon

Instructions:

Preheat the oven to 350°F (175°C).

In a bowl, mix almond flour, coconut oil, honey, and vanilla extract until combined.

Press mixture into the bottom of a greased 8x8-inch baking dish.

Top with blueberries, lemon zest, and juice.

Bake for 20-25 minutes until set.

Cool before cutting into bars.

Baked Peaches with Honey

Servings: 4   **Calories:** 100 per serving

Ingredients:

4 ripe peaches, halved and pitted

2 tablespoons honey

1 teaspoon ground cinnamon

Instructions:

Preheat the oven to 375°F (190°C).

Place peach halves in a baking dish.

Drizzle with honey and sprinkle with cinnamon.

Bake for 20-25 minutes until tender.

Serve warm.

Pear and Almond Crisp

Servings: 6   **Calories:** 150 per serving

Ingredients:

4 ripe pears, peeled and sliced

1/4 cup almond flour

1/4 cup rolled oats

2 tablespoons honey

2 tablespoons coconut oil, melted

1 teaspoon ground cinnamon

Instructions:

Preheat the oven to 350°F (175°C).

In a baking dish, layer sliced pears.

In a bowl, mix almond flour, oats, honey, coconut oil, and cinnamon.

Sprinkle mixture over pears.

Bake for 25-30 minutes until topping is golden brown.

Serve warm.

7. MEAL PLANNING AND PREP

Managing diverticulitis through diet involves strategic meal planning and preparation. This ensures that your meals are nutritious, easy to digest, and aligned with the dietary phases of diverticulitis. Here's a guide to help you plan and prepare your meals efficiently.

Weekly Meal Planning

Step 1: Plan Your Meals

Use a weekly planner to schedule your meals and snacks.

Ensure a balanced intake of proteins, carbohydrates, and healthy fats.

Incorporate a variety of foods to keep meals interesting and nutritious.

Step 2: Grocery Shopping

Create a shopping list based on your meal plan.

Stick to the list to avoid unnecessary purchases.

Choose fresh, whole foods over processed items.

30-DAY MEAL PLAN

Week 1

Day 1

Breakfast: Greek Yogurt with Berries and Honey

Snack: Apple Slices with Almond Butter

Lunch: Lentil and Sweet Potato Curry

Snack: Cottage Cheese and Pineapple

Dinner: Lemon Garlic Baked Tilapia with Steamed Broccoli

Day 2

Breakfast: Oatmeal with Blueberries and Honey

Snack: Hummus and Veggie Sticks

Lunch: Quinoa Tabbouleh

Snack: Greek Yogurt and Cucumber Dip

Dinner: Chicken and Broccoli Alfredo

Day 3

Breakfast: Smoothie with Spinach, Banana, and Almond Milk

Snack: Roasted Chickpeas

Lunch: Beef and Vegetable Stir-Fry with Brown Rice

Snack: Baked Zucchini Chips

Dinner: Spaghetti Squash with Marinara Sauce

Day 4

Breakfast: Whole Wheat Toast with Avocado and Poached Egg

Snack: Cucumber and Avocado Salad

Lunch: Greek Salad with Grilled Chicken

Snack: Tomato and Mozzarella Salad

Dinner: Herb-Crusted Pork Tenderloin with Roasted Cauliflower

Day 5

Breakfast: Quinoa Porridge with Apple and Cinnamon

Snack: Guacamole with Baked Pita Chips

Lunch: Chicken and Rice Stuffed Zucchini

Snack: Berry and Spinach Smoothie

Dinner: Lemon Herb Salmon with Quinoa and Asparagus

Day 6

Breakfast: Greek Yogurt with Berries and Honey

Snack: Spinach and Feta Stuffed Mushrooms

Lunch: Turkey and Avocado Wrap

Snack: Apple Slices with Almond Butter

Dinner: Baked Falafel with Tahini Sauce and Steamed Green Beans

Day 7

Breakfast: Scrambled Eggs with Spinach and Tomatoes

Snack: Greek Yogurt and Cucumber Dip with Veggie Sticks

Lunch: Black Bean and Quinoa Stuffed Bell Peppers

Snack: Steamed Asparagus with Lemon

Dinner: Roasted Chicken Thighs with Sweet Potato Fries

Day 8
Breakfast: Whole Wheat Pancakes with Maple Syrup

Snack: Carrot and Ginger Soup

Lunch: Lentil and Sweet Potato Curry

Snack: Cottage Cheese and Pineapple

Dinner: Lemon Garlic Baked Tilapia with Steamed Broccoli

Day 9
Breakfast: Greek Yogurt with Berries and Honey

Snack: Baked Zucchini Chips

Lunch: Quinoa Tabbouleh

Snack: Guacamole with Baked Pita Chips

Dinner: Chicken and Broccoli Alfredo

Day 10
Breakfast: Smoothie with Spinach, Banana, and Almond Milk

Snack: Roasted Chickpeas

Lunch: Beef and Vegetable Stir-Fry with Brown Rice

Snack: Greek Yogurt and Cucumber Dip

Dinner: Spaghetti Squash with Marinara Sauce

Day 11
Breakfast: Whole Wheat Toast with Avocado and Poached Egg

Snack: Cucumber and Avocado Salad

Lunch: Greek Salad with Grilled Chicken

Snack: Tomato and Mozzarella Salad

Dinner: Herb-Crusted Pork Tenderloin with Roasted Cauliflower

Day 12
Breakfast: Oatmeal with Blueberries and Honey

Snack: Hummus and Veggie Sticks

Lunch: Chicken and Rice Stuffed Zucchini

Snack: Berry and Spinach Smoothie

Dinner: Lemon Herb Salmon with Quinoa and Asparagus

Day 13
Breakfast: Greek Yogurt with Berries and Honey

Snack: Spinach and Feta Stuffed Mushrooms

Lunch: Turkey and Avocado Wrap

Snack: Apple Slices with Almond Butter

Dinner: Baked Falafel with Tahini Sauce and Steamed Green Beans

Day 14
Breakfast: Scrambled Eggs with Spinach and Tomatoes

Snack: Greek Yogurt and Cucumber Dip with Veggie Sticks

Lunch: Black Bean and Quinoa Stuffed Bell Peppers

Snack: Steamed Asparagus with Lemon

Dinner: Roasted Chicken Thighs with Sweet Potato Fries

Day 15
Breakfast: Greek Yogurt with Berries and Honey

Snack: Apple Slices with Almond Butter

Lunch: Lentil and Sweet Potato Curry

Snack: Cottage Cheese and Pineapple

Dinner: Lemon Garlic Baked Tilapia with Steamed Broccoli

Day 16
Breakfast: Oatmeal with Blueberries and Honey

Snack: Hummus and Veggie Sticks

Lunch: Quinoa Tabbouleh

Snack: Greek Yogurt and Cucumber Dip

Dinner: Chicken and Broccoli Alfredo

Day 17
Breakfast: Smoothie with Spinach, Banana, and Almond Milk

Snack: Roasted Chickpeas

Lunch: Beef and Vegetable Stir-Fry with Brown Rice

Snack: Baked Zucchini Chips

Dinner: Spaghetti Squash with Marinara Sauce

Day 18
Breakfast: Whole Wheat Toast with Avocado and Poached Egg

Snack: Cucumber and Avocado Salad

Lunch: Greek Salad with Grilled Chicken

Snack: Tomato and Mozzarella Salad

Dinner: Herb-Crusted Pork Tenderloin with Roasted Cauliflower

Day 19
Breakfast: Quinoa Porridge with Apple and Cinnamon

Snack: Guacamole with Baked Pita Chips

Lunch: Chicken and Rice Stuffed Zucchini

Snack: Berry and Spinach Smoothie

Dinner: Lemon Herb Salmon with Quinoa and Asparagus

Day 20
Breakfast: Greek Yogurt with Berries and Honey

Snack: Spinach and Feta Stuffed Mushrooms

Lunch: Turkey and Avocado Wrap

Snack: Apple Slices with Almond Butter

Dinner: Baked Falafel with Tahini Sauce and Steamed Green Beans

Day 21
Breakfast: Scrambled Eggs with Spinach and Tomatoes

Snack: Greek Yogurt and Cucumber Dip with Veggie Sticks

Lunch: Black Bean and Quinoa Stuffed Bell Peppers

Snack: Steamed Asparagus with Lemon

Dinner: Roasted Chicken Thighs with Sweet Potato Fries

Day 22

Breakfast: Whole Wheat Pancakes with Maple Syrup

Snack: Carrot and Ginger Soup

Lunch: Lentil and Sweet Potato Curry

Snack: Cottage Cheese and Pineapple

Dinner: Lemon Garlic Baked Tilapia with Steamed Broccoli

Day 23

Breakfast: Greek Yogurt with Berries and Honey

Snack: Baked Zucchini Chips

Lunch: Quinoa Tabbouleh

Snack: Guacamole with Baked Pita Chips

Dinner: Chicken and Broccoli Alfredo

Day 24

Breakfast: Smoothie with Spinach, Banana, and Almond Milk

Snack: Roasted Chickpeas

Lunch: Beef and Vegetable Stir-Fry with Brown Rice

Snack: Greek Yogurt and Cucumber Dip

Dinner: Spaghetti Squash with Marinara Sauce

Day 25

Breakfast: Whole Wheat Toast with Avocado and Poached Egg

Snack: Cucumber and Avocado Salad

Lunch: Greek Salad with Grilled Chicken

Snack: Tomato and Mozzarella Salad

Dinner: Herb-Crusted Pork Tenderloin with Roasted Cauliflower

Day 26

Breakfast: Oatmeal with Blueberries and Honey

Snack: Hummus and Veggie Sticks

Lunch: Chicken and Rice Stuffed Zucchini

Snack: Berry and Spinach Smoothie

Dinner: Lemon Herb Salmon with Quinoa and Asparagus

Day 27

Breakfast: Greek Yogurt with Berries and Honey

Snack: Spinach and Feta Stuffed Mushrooms

Lunch: Turkey and Avocado Wrap

Snack: Apple Slices with Almond Butter

Dinner: Baked Falafel with Tahini Sauce and Steamed Green Beans

Day 28

Breakfast: Scrambled Eggs with Spinach and Tomatoes

Snack: Greek Yogurt and Cucumber Dip with Veggie Sticks

Lunch: Black Bean and Quinoa Stuffed Bell Peppers

Snack: Steamed Asparagus with Lemon

Dinner: Roasted Chicken Thighs with Sweet Potato Fries

Day 29

Breakfast: Greek Yogurt with Berries and Honey

Snack: Apple Slices with Almond Butter

Lunch: Lentil and Sweet Potato Curry

Snack: Cottage Cheese and Pineapple

Dinner: Lemon Garlic Baked Tilapia with Steamed Broccoli

Day 30

Breakfast: Oatmeal with Blueberries and Honey

Snack: Hummus and Veggie Sticks

Lunch: Quinoa Tabbouleh

Snack: Greek Yogurt and Cucumber Dip

Dinner: Chicken and Broccoli Alfredo

CONCLUSION

Living with diverticulitis doesn't mean you have to compromise on taste or variety. With the recipes and meal plans in this cookbook, you can enjoy delicious meals while managing your symptoms. Remember to listen to your body, stay hydrated, and consult with your healthcare provider to tailor your diet to your specific needs.

Thank you for choosing the "The Simple Diverticulitis Cookbook 101." May it guide you to a healthier, happier, and more comfortable life. Bon appétit!

MEASUREMENT AND CONVERSIONS

CUPS	OZ	G	TBSP	TSP	ML
1	8	225	16	48	250
3/4	6	170	12	36	175
2/3	5	140	11	32	150
1/2	4	115	8	24	125
1/3	3	70	5	16	70
1/4	2	60	4	12	60
1/8	1	30	2	6	30
1/16	1/2	15	1	3	15

250°F	300°F	325°F	350°F	400°F	450°F
120°C	150°F	160°C	175°C	200°C	230°C

ABOUT THE AUTHOR

Adeola Ganiu is passionate writer about empowering people to lead active healthy lifestyles by teaching them the personalized skills they need to fuel themselves with whole foods while maintaining a healthy life balance.

RECIPE INDEX